Vegan Recipes in 30 Minutes

The latest Vegan recipes for busy people, this guide will help you save time and denier by eating healthy and wholesome foods.

Bruce Mitchell

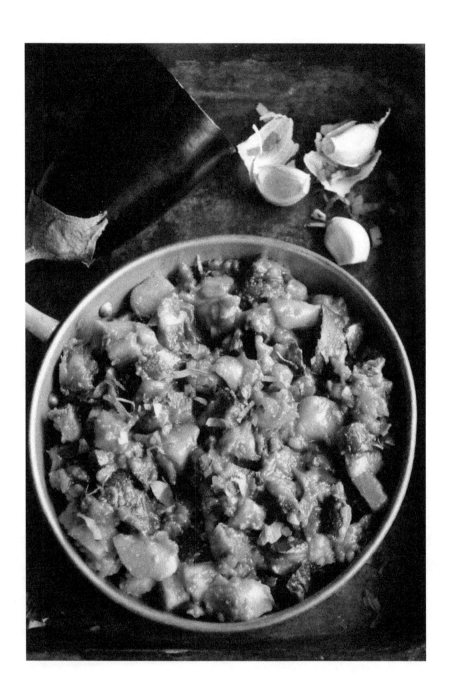

Table of Contents

INTRODUCTION 7

ENTRÉES 14

    BLT PANINI WITH EGGPLANT "BACON" 14

    VEGGIE HUMMUS WRAPS 17

    QUICK AND EASY CURRY 20

    CHICKPEA AVOCADO SALAD SANDWICHES 22

    ITALIAN "MEATBALL" SUBS 24

    SUNDRIED TOMATO AND MUSHROOM PENNE PASTA 27

FRUIT SALAD RECIPES 31

    AMBROSIA WITH PINEAPPLE 31

    TROPICAL FRUIT SALAD 33

    FALL FRUIT WITH CREAMY DRESSING 34

    SUMMERTIME FRUIT SALAD 36

    CHERRY BERRY SALAD 38

    FRUIT SALAD WITH SWEET LIME DRESSING 40

    ASIAN FRUIT SALAD 42

    MIMOSA SALAD 44

    HONEY LIME QUINOA FRUIT SALAD 45

GRAINS AND BEANS 46

    VEGGIE BARLEY BOWL 46

    INDIAN LENTIL DAHL 48

    KALE AND SWEET POTATO QUINOA 50

    BROWN RICE WITH MUSHROOMS 53

    VEGGIE PAELLA 55

    VEGETABLE AND WILD RICE PILAF 57

    BROWN RICE WITH SPICED VEGETABLES 59

    SPICED TOMATO BROWN RICE 61

    NOODLE AND RICE PILAF 63

    EASY MILLET LOAF 65

    WALNUT-OAT BURGERS 67

    SPICY BEANS AND RICE 69

    BLACK-EYED PEAS AND CORN SALAD 71

    INDIAN TOMATO AND GARBANZO STEW 73

    SIMPLE BAKED NAVY BEANS 75

VINEGARY BLACK BEANS...77
SPICED LENTIL BURGERS 79
PECAN-MAPLE GRANOLA 81
BEAN AND SUMMER SQUASH SAUTÉ...83
PEPPERY BLACK BEANS 85
WALNUT, COCONUT, AND OAT GRANOLA..87
RITZY FAVA BEAN RATATOUILLE 89
PEPPERS AND BLACK BEANS WITH BROWN RICE............................91
BLACK-EYED PEA, BEET, AND CARROT STEW 93
KOSHARI 95

DRINKS **98**

CHOCOLATEY BANANA SHAKE..98
FRUITY TOFU SMOOTHIE 100
GREEN FRUITY SMOOTHIE 102
PROTEIN LATTE 104
HEALTH BOOSTING JUICES 105
THAI ICED TEA...107
HOT CHOCOLATE...109
CHAI AND CHOCOLATE MILKSHAKE...110
COLORFUL INFUSED WATER...112
HIBISCUS TEA 114
LEMON AND ROSEMARY ICED TEA 116
LAVENDER AND MINT ICED TEA..118

CONCLUSION...**120**

5

INTRODUCTION

The Merriam Webster Dictionary defines a vegetarian as one contains a wholly of vegetables, grains, nuts, fruits, and sometimes eggs or dairy products. It has also been described as a plant-based diet that relies wholly on plant-foods such as fruits, whole grains, herbs, vegetables, nuts, seeds, and spices. Whatever way you want to look at it, the reliance wholly on plants stands the vegetarian diet out from other types of diets. People become vegetarians for different reasons. Some take up this nutritional plan for medical or health reasons. For example, people suffering from cardiovascular diseases or who stand the risk of developing such diseases are usually advised to refrain from meat generally and focus on a plant-based diet, rich in fruits and vegetables. Some other individuals become vegetarians for religious or ethical reasons.

On this side of the spectrum are Hinduism, Jainism, Buddhism, Seventh-Day Adventists, and some other religions. It is believed that being a vegetarian is part of being holy and keeping with the ideals of non-violence. For ethical reasons, some animal rights activists are also vegetarians based on the belief that animals have rights and should not be slaughtered for food. Yet another set of persons become vegetarians based on food preference. Such individuals are naturally more disposed to a plant-based diet and find meat and other related food products less pleasurable. Some refrain from meat as a protest against climate change. This is based on the environmental concern that rearing livestock contributes to climate change and greenhouse gas emissions and the waste of natural resources in maintaining such livestock. People are usually very quick to throw words around without exactly knowing what a Vegetarian Diet means. In the same vein, the term "vegetarian" has become a popular one in recent years. What exactly does this word connote, and what does it not mean?

At its simplest, the word "vegetarian" refers to a person who refrains from eating meat, beef, pork, lard, chicken, or even fish. Depending on the kind of vegetarian it is, however, a vegetarian could either eat or exclude from his diet animal products. Animal products would refer to foods such as eggs, dairy products, and even honey! A vegetarian diet would, therefore, refer to the nutritional plan of the void of meat. It is the eating lifestyle of individuals who depend on plant-based foods for nutrition. It excludes animal products, particularly meat - a common denominator for all kinds of Vegetarians - from their diets. A vegetarian could also be defined as a meal plan that consists of foods coming majorly from plants to the exclusion of meat, poultry, and seafood.

This kind of Vegetarian diet usually contains no animal protein.

It is completely understandable from the discussion so far that the term "vegetarian" is more or less a blanket term covering different plant-based diets. While reliance majorly on plant foods is consistent in all the different types of vegetarians, they have some underlying differences. The different types of vegetarians are discussed below:

Veganism: This is undoubtedly the strictest type of vegetarian diet. Vegans exclude the any animal product. It goes as far as avoiding animal-derived ingredients contained in processed foods. Whether its meat, poultry products like eggs, dairy products inclusive of milk, honey, or even gelatin, they all are excluded from the vegans.

Some vegans go beyond nutrition and go as far as refusing to wear clothes that contain animal products. This means such vegans do not wear leather, wool, or silk.

Lacto-vegetarian: This kind of vegetarian excludes meat, fish, and poultry. However, it allows the inclusion of dairy products such as milk, yogurt, cheese, and butter. The hint is perhaps in the name since Lacto means milk in Latin.

Ovo-Vegetarian: Meat and dairy products are excluded under this diet, but eggs could be consumed. Ovo means egg.

Lacto-Ovo Vegetarian: This appears to be the hybrid of the Ovo Vegetarian and the Lacto-Vegetarian. This is the most famous type of vegetarian diet and is usually what comes to mind when people think of the Vegetarian. This type of Vegetarian bars all kinds of meat but allows for the consumption of eggs and dairy products.

Pollotarian: This vegetarian allows the consumption of chicken.

Pescatarian: This refers to the vegetarian that consumes fish. More people are beginning to subscribe to this kind of diet due to health reasons.

Flexitarian: Flexitarians are individuals who prefer plant-based foods to meat but have no problem eating meats once in a while. They are also referred to as semi-vegetarians.

Raw Vegan: This is also called the raw food and consists of a vegan that is yet to be processed and has also not been heated over 46 C. This kind of diet has its root in the belief that nutrients and minerals present in the plant diet are lost when cooked on temperature above 46 C and could also become harmful to the body.

ENTRÉES

BLT Panini with Eggplant "Bacon"

Preparation Time: 10 minutes

Cooking Time: 25 minutes

Servings: 2

Ingredients:

- Eggplant, medium – 1
- Tomato, sliced into rounds – 1
- Cucumber, medium, sliced into rounds - .5
- Arugula lettuce - .5 cup
- Vegan mayonnaise – 2 tablespoons
- Ciabatta buns – 2
- Tamari sauce – 1 tablespoon
- Sea salt - 1.25 teaspoon
- Maple syrup – 1 teaspoon
- Olive oil – 1 tablespoon
- Paprika, smoked – 1 teaspoon
- Black pepper, ground - .25 teaspoon

Directions:

1. Peel the eggplant, slice it into rounds, and soak it in salt water made with one teaspoon of the sea salt. Allow the eggplant to sit in the saltwater for ten minutes. Remove the eggplant from the saltwater once soaked for the ten-minute duration and then pat it dry with a clean kitchen towel.

2. In a small bowl whisk together the tamari sauce, sea salt, maple syrup, olive oil, smoked paprika, and ground black pepper.

3. Place the eggplant slices on a baking sheet. Use the combined sauce and with a pastry brush cover it over the eggplant slices on all sides. Bake the eggplant slices until tender, for about twenty minutes in a large oven preheated to a temperature of three-hundred- and seventy-five-degrees Fahrenheit.

4. Once the eggplant is done cooking prepare your panini. Begin by slicing the ciabatta rolls in half. Spread the inside of the rolls with vegan mayonnaise before topping with the eggplant "bacon," tomato, cucumber, and lastly the

arugula. Close the sandwich with the top half of the rolls.

5. Wrap the sandwiches in aluminum foil before placing them in a panini grill. However, if you do not have a panini grill, you can do this in a large skillet by weighing down the sandwich with a heavy pan, such as a small cast iron pan.

6. Allow the sandwiches to grill until warm and crispy, about three to four minutes. Enjoy the sandwich immediately, or leave it in the aluminum foil to take on-the-go.

Nutrition: Number of Calories in Individual **Servings:** 364 Protein Grams: 10   Fat Grams: 14 Total Carbohydrates Grams: 51 Net Carbohydrates Grams: 41

Veggie Hummus Wraps

Preparation Time: 10 minutes

Cooking Time: 6 minutes

Servings: 2

Ingredients:

- Zucchini, peeled, sliced lengthwise into .25-inch-thick strips – 1
- Sea salt - .5 teaspoon
- Tomato, sliced – 1
- Kale, chopped – 1 cup
- Red onion, sliced - .125 cup
- Avocado, sliced – 1
- Olive oil – 1 tablespoon
- Black pepper, ground - .25 teaspoon
- Apple cider vinegar – 2 teaspoons
- Water – 1 tablespoon
- Hummus - .25 cup
- Whole-wheat tortillas, large – 2

Directions:

1. Heat a large non-stick skillet or grill pan on the stove over medium heat. Meanwhile, coat the

sliced zucchini with the olive oil, ground black pepper, and sea salt.

2. Place the seasoned zucchini on the preheated pan and let it cook on the first side for three minutes, flip it over, and cook for an additional two minutes. Remove the zucchini from the heat of the stove and set it aside.

3. Set the whole-wheat tortillas in the hot pan and allow them to toast for a minute. You want the tortillas to be lightly toasted, warm, and easy to wrap without tearing.

4. Combine the apple cider vinegar and water, then toss the avocado in the mixture. This will help prevent the avocado from browning. Drain off any excess liquid.

5. Divide the ingredients in half, so that you can fill both tortillas with an even amount of ingredients. To prepare spread the hummus down the center of the warm tortilla, top with the zucchini, tomato, red onion, kale, and avocado.

6. Wrap in the ends of the tortillas and then tightly wrap the sides around the filling. By folding it

this way, you will prevent the filling from falling out. Serve immediately or store in the fridge until lunchtime.

Nutrition: Number of Calories in Individual **Servings:** 438 Protein Grams: 9 Fat Grams: 28 Total Carbohydrates Grams: 40 Net Carbohydrates Grams: 36

Quick and Easy Curry

Preparation Time: 10 minutes

Cooking Time: 25 minutes

Servings: 4

Ingredients:

- Bell peppers, red, thinly sliced – 2
- Chickpeas, cooked, liquid drained off – 2.5 cups or a 19 ounce can
- Broccoli florets, roughly chopped – 4 cups
- Onion, diced – 1
- Light coconut milk – 14 ounces
- Maple syrup – 1 teaspoon
- Sea salt – 1 teaspoon
- Tamari sauce – 1 tablespoon
- Garlic, minced – 4 cloves
- Cumin – 1 tablespoon
- Curry powder – 1 tablespoon
- Black pepper, ground - .25 teaspoon
- Water - .25 cup

Directions:

1. Place all of the vegetables and the water into a large non-stick skillet and allow them to cook together over a temperature of medium-high heat for three minutes.

2. Add the remaining ingredients and continue to cook the curry for seven to eight minutes, until the vegetables are tender but still have a little bite. You don't want to overcook the vegetables until they become mush, as they are best with their texture intact.

3. Remove the curry from the heat, give it a good stir, and serve it with your favorite cooked grains or pasta.

Nutrition: Number of Calories in Individual **Servings:** 342 Protein Grams: 15 Fat Grams: 6 Total Carbohydrates Grams: 52 Net Carbohydrates Grams: 39

Chickpea Avocado Salad Sandwiches

Preparation Time: 10 minutes

Cooking Time: 0 minutes

Servings: 4

Ingredients:

- Chickpeas, liquid drained, rinsed – 15 ounce can (1.5 cups)
- Red onion, diced - .5 cup
- Lemon juice – 2 tablespoons
- Cilantro, fresh, chopped - .25 cup
- Thyme, fresh, chopped – 1 tablespoon
- Avocado, diced – 1 cup
- Red grapes, sliced in half - .5 cup
- Celery, finely sliced - .25 cup
- Sea salt – 1 teaspoon
- Whole-wheat bread – 6 slices

Directions:

1. Place the drained and rinse chickpeas and the diced avocado in a medium-sized bowl for the purpose of mixing. Using a fork or potato

masher smash the ingredients together until you form a chunky and creamy mixture. You can do this to your preference, either leaving the chickpeas mostly whole or smashing them until they are mostly creamy.

2. Add the red onion, lemon juice, fresh cilantro, fresh thyme, red grapes, celery, and sea salt to the bowl and stir all of the ingredients together until combined.

3. Divide the chickpea salad mixture between three slices of bread, and then top it off with the remaining three slices. Of course, you can always save the mixture in the fridge for another day, and then assemble your sandwiches on the day you plan to consume them. Don't fill your sandwiches with the filling more than a day ahead of time, as you don't want soggy bread.

Nutrition: Number of Calories in Individual **Servings:** 486 Protein Grams: 16 Fat Grams: 13 Total Carbohydrates Grams: 80 Net Carbohydrates Grams: 65

Italian "Meatball" Subs

Preparation Time: 5 minutes

Cooking Time: 55 minutes

Servings: 4

Ingredients:

- Chickpeas, liquid drained, rinsed – 15 ounces (1.5 cups)
- Bread crumbs - .25 cup
- Flaxseed, ground – 1.5 tablespoons
- Water, warm – .25 cup
- Nutritional yeast – 2 tablespoons
- Italian seasoning - .5 teaspoon
- Sea salt - .5 teaspoon
- Garlic powder – 2 teaspoons
- Sub rolls, medium – 3
- Vegan mozzarella cheese, shredded (such as Daiya or homemade) – .75 cup
- Marinara sauce – 1 cup

Directions:

1. Preheat your large oven to a temperature of Fahrenheit four-hundred and twenty-five

degrees. Meanwhile, assemble your chickpea "meatballs."

2. In a medium-sized bowl for the purpose of mixing whisk together the warm water and flaxseed until all of the clumps are gone. Allow it to sit for five minutes.

3. Meanwhile, place the chickpeas in the food processor with the standard blade and pulse them until they are finely ground with no whole beans remaining. Place the chickpea meal into the bowl with the flaxseed mixture.

4. Add the sea salt, bread crumbs, Italian seasoning, nutritional yeast, and garlic powder to the chickpea and flaxseed bowl, combining the ingredients together completely with a spoon.

5. Using a mini cookie scoop or tablespoon measure out evenly sized "meatballs" with the mixture, rolling them into balls in the palms of your hands. Place these prepared meatballs on a baking sheet lined with kitchen parchment and allow them to cook in the hot oven for fifteen

minutes before turning the pan around and cooking for an additional fifteen minutes.

6. Reduce the oven temperature to that of Fahrenheit four-hundred degrees.

7. Place the cooked meatballs in a large saucepan and add in the marinara sauce, heating it on a stove burner set to medium-low heat until the sauce is hot all the way through. Occasionally stir the chickpea meatballs in the marinara sauce so that they are evenly coated.

8. Fill the sub rolls with the meatballs and sauce, top them with the dairy-free cheese, and place them in the hot often on the baking sheet for fifteen minutes, or until the dairy-free cheese is melted and the bread is warm. Enjoy the subs hot and fresh from the oven.

Nutrition: Number of Calories in Individual **Servings:** 376 Protein Grams: 16 Fat Grams: 9 Total Carbohydrates Grams: 57 Net Carbohydrates Grams: 67

Sundried Tomato and Mushroom Penne Pasta

Preparation Time: 10 minutes

Cooking Time: 20 minutes

Servings: 4

Ingredients:

- Penne pasta, uncooked – 250 grams
- Corn starch – 2.5 tablespoons
- Olive oil – 4 teaspoons
- Garlic, minced – 6 cloves
- Sundried tomatoes, drained from the oil - .75 cup
- Soy milk (or almond), unsweetened – 2 cups
- Onion, diced – 1
- Oregano, dried -.5 teaspoon
- Nutritional yeast – 1 tablespoon
- Sea salt – 1 teaspoon
- Mushrooms, sliced – 1.5 cups
- Chili flakes – 1 teaspoon
- Black pepper, ground - .25 teaspoon

Directions:

1. Place the pasta in a large pot of salted boiling water and cook it according to the individual brand's instructions, but don't cook it quite all the way. Instead, allow the pasta to remain slightly under-cooked, as you will finish cooking it later on. Drain the pasta, reserving the pasta water.

2. Place a large frying pan on the large burner of your stove surface and set it to a medium temperature. Add in three teaspoons of the olive oil and the mushrooms, cooking for two minutes before adding in the garlic. Cook for an additional two minutes, until the mushrooms, are tender, and the garlic is fragrant.

3. Remove the mushrooms and garlic from the skillet and set them aside.

4. Add the corn starch, sea salt, and half of the soy milk into the hot skillet. Use a whisk to make sure that there are no clumps of corn starch and that the sauce is smooth. Once thickened, add the remaining soy milk and whisk again.

5. Into a blender pour the hot sauce mixture, nutritional yeast, half of the sundried tomatoes,

and .33 cup of the hot pasta water. Blend the
mixture on medium to high speed, being sure
that it does not overflow from the heat buildup.
Once blended smooth set the sauce aside.

6. Rinse out the previously used skillet and then
    add in the remaining teaspoon of olive oil. Chop
    the remaining sundried tomatoes and add them
    into the skillet along with the diced onion,
    allowing them to cook for three minutes until the
    onion becomes translucent. Add in the dried
    oregano and chili flakes, cooking the skillet for
    an additional minute until fragrant. If the
    ingredients begin to stick to the skillet simply
    add in a small amount of the reserved pasta
    water.

7. Add the prepared sauce into the skillet with the
    onion and sundried tomatoes, stirring all of the
    ingredients together. Add in the pasta, coating it
    in the sauce and adding any pasta water if you
    need to loosen the sauce.

8. Continue to cook the ingredients together until
    the pasta is al dente and then serve.

Nutrition: Number of Calories in Individual

Servings: 350 Protein Grams: 14 Fat Grams: 8

Total Carbohydrates Grams: 55 Net Carbohydrates

Grams: 50

FRUIT SALAD RECIPES

Ambrosia with Pineapple

Preparation Time: 30 Minutes

Cooking Time: 15 Minutes

Servings: 4

Ingredients:

- Orange zest, two teaspoons
- Tofu, soft, pureed, one half cup
- Orange juice, three tablespoons
- Lemon juice, one third cup
- Cornstarch, one tablespoon
- Coconut, unsweetened shredded, one half cup
- Grapes, one cup
- Sugar, three tablespoons
- Strawberries, sliced, one cup
- Orange slices, one cup
- Apples, fresh sliced, one cup
- Pineapple, fresh chopped, one cup

Directions:

1. Use a large-sized bowl to assemble the fruits together and put it in the refrigerator.
2. In a small saucepan, mix together the lemon juice with the cornstarch and keep stirring until they are well mixed.
3. Add in the orange juice and the sugar and place the saucepan over medium-high heat. Cook the mix for five to ten minutes while the mixture gets thicker. Keep stirring constantly.
4. When the mixture is thick, then take the saucepan off of the heat and let it get completely cool.
5. When the mixture in the saucepan has cooled completely, then blends in the orange zest and the pureed tofu.
6. Allow this bowl of mix to rest in the refrigerator for one hour until it becomes chilled. Pour the dressing over the fruit before serving.

Nutrition: Calories: 257 Protein: 8g Fat: 8g Carbs: 44g

Tropical Fruit Salad

Preparation Time: 10 Minutes

Cooking Time: 0 Minutes

Servings: 2

Ingredients:

- Lime juice, one tablespoon
- Kiwi, two
- Dragon fruit, one half of one
- Strawberries, twelve
- Mango, one half of one

Directions:

1. Peel the fruits and chop them into bite-sized pieces. Dump all of the fruit chunks into a large-sized mixing bowl.

2. Drizzle the lime juice over the fruit and toss the fruit gently to coat all of the pieces with the juice. Serve immediately

Nutrition: Calories: 154 Protein: 2g Fat: 1g Carbs: 37g

Fall Fruit with Creamy Dressing

Preparation Time: 25 Minutes

Cooking Time: 0 Minutes

Servings: 4

Ingredients:

Salad

- Pumpkin, raw, shredded, one half cup
- Pomegranate seeds, one half cup
- Grapes, one cup
- Apples, three, cored and cubed

Creamy Dressing

- Cinnamon, one teaspoon
- Lemon juice, one tablespoon
- Almond yogurt, one half cup

Directions:

1. Mix together all of the listed Ingredients for the dressing.

2. In a large-sized bowl, toss the dressing with the shredded raw pumpkin, pomegranate seeds, apples, and the dressing. Serve immediately.

Nutrition: Calories: 161 Protein: 3g Fat: 1g

Carbs: 40g

Summertime Fruit Salad

Preparation Time: 15 Minutes

Cooking Time: 0 Minutes

Servings: 6

Ingredients:

- Balsamic vinegar, two teaspoons
- Lemon juice, two tablespoons
- Mint, fresh chopped, one tablespoon
- Blueberries, one cup
- Peaches, fresh, three, peeled and sliced thin
- Strawberries, one pound, cleaned and sliced thin

Directions:

1. Mix together in a medium-sized serving bowl the basil, blueberries, peaches, and strawberries. In a small-sized bowl, mix together the balsamic vinegar and the lemon juice.

2. Pour the liquid dressing over the mixed fruit and toss gently to coat all of the pieces of fruit with the dressing.

3. Serve immediately or keep the salad covered in the refrigerator for no longer than two days.

Nutrition: Calories: 91 Protein: 1g Fat: 6g Carbs: 22g

Cherry Berry Salad

Preparation Time: 10 Minutes

Cooking Time: 0 Minutes

Servings: 6

Ingredients:

- Lemon juice, three tablespoons
- Cardamom, one quarter teaspoon
- Cinnamon, one half teaspoon
- Mint, fresh, three tablespoons
- Blackberries, one cup
- Blueberries, one cup
- Raspberries, one cup
- Cherries, seeded, cut in half, one cup
- Strawberries, cleaned, two cups quartered

Directions:

1. In a small-sized bowl, mix the spices and the lemon juice together well. In a medium-sized bowl, mix the fruits together with the lemon juice and mint mixture.

2. Toss the fruits gently but thoroughly to coat all of the pieces. This will store well in the refrigerator for two to three days.

Nutrition: Calories: 113 Protein: 1g Fat: 1g Carbs: 27g

Fruit Salad with Sweet Lime Dressing

Preparation Time: 15 Minutes

Cooking Time: 0 Minutes

Servings: 9

Ingredients:

Salad

- Mint, fresh chopped, one cup
- Lime juice, two tablespoons
- Kiwi, five, peeled and sliced
- Mangoes, two, peeled and chopped
- Green grapes, one cup cut in half
- Blackberries, one cup
- Blueberries, one cup
- Strawberries, one cup sliced

Sweet Lime Dressing

- Powdered sugar, two tablespoons
- Lime juice, two tablespoons

Directions:

1. Mix together until smooth in a small-sized bowl the powdered sugar and the lime juice.

2. Mix together in a large-sized bowl the fruits, then pour on the dressing and gently toss all of the fruits together well to coat all of the pieces.

3. This will stay good in the refrigerator for no more than one day.

Nutrition: Calories: 50 Protein: 1g Fat: 1g Carbs: 12g

Asian Fruit Salad

Preparation Time: 30 Minutes

Cooking Time: 0 Minutes

Servings: 8

Ingredients:

- Passion fruit, one-half cup (about six of the fruit)
- Papaya, one chopped
- Pineapple, one cup chunked
- Oranges, two separated into segments
- Star fruit, three sliced thin
- Mangoes, two large, peeled and chunked
- Mint, fresh, one-third cup chopped coarse
- Lime juice, one third cup
- Lime zest, one tablespoon
- Ginger, ground, one tablespoon
- Vanilla extract, one tablespoon
- Brown sugar, one half cup
- Water, four cups

Directions:

1. Mix the water and the sugar together in a medium-sized saucepan and put it over a medium to high heat until the sugar is dissolved.
2. Let this simmer for five minutes over a very low heat, so the sugar does not burn. Add in the vanilla extract and the ginger and stir well.
3. Let this cook for ten more minutes. Let the mix cool off the heat until it is room temperature, and then add in the mint, juice, and zest.
4. During the time the sauce is cooling mix together the remainder of the Ingredients in a large-sized bowl.
5. Pour the syrup mixture over the fruit in the bowl and mix gently to coat all pieces with the sauce.
6. Put the bowl in the refrigerator until the fruit is cold then serve.

Nutrition: Calories: 220 Protein: 3g Fat: 1g Carbs: 56g

Mimosa Salad

Preparation Time: 10 Minutes

Cooking Time: 0 Minutes

Servings: 8

Ingredients:

- Mint, fresh, one half cup
- Orange juice, one half cup
- Pineapple, one cup cut into small pieces
- Strawberries, one cup cut into quarters
- Blueberries, one cup
- Blackberries, one cup
- Kiwi, three peeled and sliced

Directions:

1. In a large-sized bowl, mix all of the fruits together and then top with the orange juice and the fresh mint.
2. Toss gently together all of the fruit until they are well mixed.

Nutrition: Calories: 215 Protein: 3g Fat: 1g Carbs: 49g

Honey Lime Quinoa Fruit Salad

Preparation Time: 20 Minutes

Cooking Time: 0 Minutes

Servings: 6

Ingredients:

- Basil, chopped, one tablespoon
- Lime juice, two tablespoons
- Mango, diced, one cup
- Blueberries, one cup
- Blackberries, one cup
- Strawberries, sliced, one and one half cup
- Quinoa, cooked, one cup

Directions:

1. In a large-sized bowl, mix the fruits with the cooked quinoa and mix well.
2. Drizzle on the lime juice and add the chopped basil and mix the fruit gently but thoroughly to coat all of the pieces.

Nutrition: Calories: 246 Protein: 7g Fat: 1g Carbs: 44g

GRAINS AND BEANS

Veggie Barley Bowl

Preparation Time: 10 minutes

Cooking Time: 1 hour 11 minutes

Servings: 8

Ingredients:

- 1 cup barley
- 3 cups low-sodium vegetable broth
- 2 cups sliced mushrooms
- 2 cups broccoli florets
- 1 cup snow peas, trimmed
- ½ cup sliced scallion
- ¼ cup chopped green bell pepper
- ¼ cup chopped red bell pepper
- 1 cup bean sprouts
- ¼ cup soy sauce
- ¼ cup water
- ¼ teaspoon ground ginger

—

- 1 tablespoon cornstarch, mixed with 2 tablespoons cold water

Directions:

1. In a saucepan over medium heat, place the barley and vegetable stock. Cover and cook for 1 hour.

2. Combine all the vegetables, except for the bean sprouts, in a large pot with the soy sauce, water and ginger. Cook for 5 minutes, stirring constantly.

3. Add the bean sprouts and cook, stirring, for another 5 minutes. Add the cornstarch mixture and cook for about 1 minute, stirring, or until thickened.

4. Remove from the heat. Toss the vegetables with the cooked barley.

5. Serve hot.

Nutrition: Calories: 190 Fat: 2.6g Carbs: 35.7g Protein: 5.9g Fiber: 6.9g

Indian Lentil Dahl

Preparation Time: 10 minutes

Cooking Time: 25 minutes

Servings: 6

Ingredients:

- 3 cup cooked basmati rice
- 2 tablespoons olive oil (optional)
- 6 garlic cloves, minced
- 2 yellow onions, finely diced
- 1-inch piece fresh ginger, minced
- 2 tomatoes, diced
- 2 tablespoons ground cumin
- 1 tablespoon ground coriander
- 1 tablespoon ground turmeric
- 1 tablespoon paprika
- 4 cups water
- 2 cups uncooked green lentils, rinsed
- 1 teaspoon salt (optional)

Directions:

1. In a large pot, heat the olive oil (if desired) over medium heat. Add the garlic, onions, and ginger. Cook for 3 minutes, or until onions are golden. Add the tomatoes and cook for 2 minutes more, stirring occasionally. Stir in the cumin, coriander, turmeric and paprika.

2. Add the water and lentils. Cover and bring to a boil over high heat. Once boiling, stir and reduce the heat to a simmer. Cook, covered, for 20 minutes, stirring every 5 minutes, or until the lentils are fully cooked and beginning to break down. Season with salt (if desired) and stir.

3. Divide the rice evenly among 6 meal prep containers. Add an equal portion of the dahl to each container. Let cool completely before putting on lids and refrigerating.

Nutrition: Calories: 432 Fat: 17.2g Carbs: 58.8g Protein: 10.9g Fiber: 8.9g

Kale and Sweet Potato Quinoa

Preparation Time: 10 minutes

Cooking Time: 19 minutes

Servings: 4

Ingredients:

- ¼ cup olive oil (optional)
- 1 yellow onion, diced
- 2 tablespoons ground coriander
- 2 tablespoons ground cumin
- 2 tablespoons mustard powder
- 2 tablespoons ground turmeric
- 2 teaspoons ground cinnamon
- 1 large sweet potato, diced
- 1¼ cup uncooked quinoa
- 4 cups water
- 1 bunch kale, rinsed and chopped
- Salt, to taste (optional)
- Freshly ground black pepper, to taste

Directions:

1. In a large pot, heat the oil (if desired) over medium-high heat. Add the onion and sauté for 3 minutes. Stir in the coriander, cumin, mustard powder, turmeric and cinnamon. Cook for about 1 minute, or until fragrant. Add the sweet potatoes and stir until well coated with the spices.
2. Stir in the quinoa and water. Cover with a lid and bring to a boil over high heat, stirring occasionally. Once the liquid is boiling, remove the lid and reduce the heat to medium-low. Simmer for 15 minutes.
3. Once the water is mostly absorbed and the sweet potato is cooked through, stir in the kale. Remove from the heat and cover with a lid. Let sit for 10 to 15 minutes. The residual heat will cook the kale and the quinoa will absorb the remaining water.
4. Taste and season with salt (if desired) and pepper. Divide evenly among 4 meal prep

containers and let cool completely before putting on lids and refrigerating.

Nutrition: Calories: 457 Fat: 16.2g Carbs: 67.9g Protein: 10.1g Fiber: 12.2g

Brown Rice with Mushrooms

Preparation Time: 15 minutes

Cooking Time: 20 minutes

Servings: 6 to 8

Ingredients:

- ½ pound (227 g) mushrooms, sliced
- 1 green bell pepper, chopped
- 1 onion, chopped
- 1 bunch scallions, chopped
- 2 cloves garlic, minced
- ½ cup water
- 5 cups cooked brown rice
- 1 (16-ounce / 454-g) can chopped tomatoes
- 1 (4-ounce / 113-g) can chopped green chilies
- 2 teaspoons chili powder
- 1 teaspoon ground cumin

Directions:

1. In a large pot, sauté the mushrooms, green pepper, onion, scallions, and garlic in the water for 10 minutes.
2. Stir in the remaining ingredients. Cook over low heat for about 10 minutes, or until heated through, stirring frequently.
3. Serve immediately.

Nutrition: Calories: 185 Fat: 2.6g Carbs: 34.5g Protein: 6.1g Fiber: 4.3g

Veggie Paella

Preparation Time: 15 minutes

Cooking Time: 52 to 58 minutes

Servings: 4

Ingredients:

- 1 onion, coarsely chopped
- 8 medium mushrooms, sliced
- 2 small zucchinis, cut in half, then sliced ½ inch thick
- 1 leek, rinsed and sliced
- 2 large cloves garlic, crushed
- 1 medium tomato, coarsely chopped
- 3 cups low-sodium vegetable broth
- 1¼ cups long-grain brown rice
- ½ teaspoon crushed saffron threads
- Freshly ground black pepper, to taste
- ½ cup frozen green peas
- ½ cup water
- Chopped fresh parsley, for garnish

Directions:

1. Pour the water in a large wok. Add the onion and sauté for 5 minutes, or until most of the liquid is absorbed.

2. Stir in the mushrooms, zucchini, leek, and garlic and cook for 2 to 3 minutes, or until softened slightly.

3. Add the tomato, broth, rice, saffron, and pepper. Bring to a boil. Reduce the heat and simmer, covered, for 30 minutes.

4. Add the peas and continue to cook for another 5 to 10 minutes. Remove from the heat and let rest for 10 minutes to allow any excess moisture to be absorbed.

5. Sprinkle with the parsley before serving.

Nutrition: Calories: 418 Fat: 3.9g Carbs: 83.2g Protein: 12.7g Fiber: 9.2g

Vegetable and Wild Rice Pilaf

Preparation Time: 10 minutes

Cooking Time: 48 to 49 minutes

Servings: 6

Ingredients:

- 1 potato, scrubbed and chopped
- 1 cup chopped cauliflower
- 1 cup chopped scallion
- 1 cup chopped broccoli
- 1 to 2 cloves garlic, minced
- 2 tablespoons soy sauce
- 3 cups low-sodium vegetable broth
- 1 cup long-grain brown rice
- 1/3 cup wild rice
- 2 small zucchinis, chopped
- ½ cup grated carrot
- 1/8 teaspoon sesame oil (optional)
- ¼ cup chopped fresh cilantro
- ½ cup water

Directions:

1. Bring the water to a boil in a large saucepan. Add the potato, cauliflower, scallion, broccoli and garlic and sauté for 2 to 3 minutes.
2. Add the soy sauce and cook for 1 minute. Add the vegetable broth, brown rice and wild rice. Bring to a boil. Reduce the heat, cover, and cook for 15 minutes.
3. Stir in the zucchinis. After another 15 minutes, stir in the carrot. Continue to cook for 15 minutes. Stir in the sesame oil (if desired) and cilantro.
4. Serve immediately.

Nutrition: Calories: 376 Fat: 3.6g Carbs: 74.5g Protein: 11.8g Fiber: 8.1g

Brown Rice with Spiced Vegetables

Preparation Time: 10 minutes

Cooking Time: 16 to 18 minutes

Servings: 6

Ingredients:

- 2 teaspoons grated fresh ginger
- 2 cloves garlic, crushed
- ½ cup water
- ¼ pound (113 g) green beans, trimmed and cut into 1-inch pieces
- 1 carrot, scrubbed and sliced
- ½ pound (227 g) mushrooms, sliced
- 2 zucchinis, cut in half lengthwise and sliced
- 1 bunch scallions, cut into 1-inch pieces
- 4 cups cooked brown rice
- 3 tablespoons soy sauce

Directions:

1. Place the ginger and garlic in a large pot with the water. Add the green beans and carrot and sauté for 3 minutes.

2. Add the mushrooms and sauté for another 2 minutes. Stir in the zucchini and scallions. Reduce the heat. Cover and cook for 6 to 8 minutes, or until the vegetables are tender-crisp, stirring frequently.

3. Stir in the rice and soy sauce. Cook over low heat for 5 minutes, or until heated through.

4. Serve warm.

Nutrition: Calories: 205 Fat: 3.0g Carbs: 38.0g Protein: 6.4g Fiber: 4.4 g

Spiced Tomato Brown Rice

Preparation Time: 10 minutes

Cooking Time: 15 minutes

Servings: 4 to 6

Ingredients:

- 1 onion, diced

- 1 green bell pepper, diced

- 3 cloves garlic, minced

- ¼ cup water

- 15 to 16 ounces (425 to 454g) tomatoes, chopped

- 1 tablespoon chili powder

- 2 teaspoons ground cumin

- 1 teaspoon dried basil

- ½ teaspoon Parsley Patch seasoning, general blend

- ¼ teaspoon cayenne

- 2 cups cooked brown rice

Directions:

1. Combine the onion, green pepper, garlic and water in a saucepan over medium heat. Cook for about 5 minutes, stirring constantly, or until softened.
2. Add the tomatoes and seasonings. Cook for another 5 minutes. Stir in the cooked rice. Cook for another 5 minutes to allow the flavors to blend.
3. Serve immediately.

Nutrition: Calories: 107 Fat: 1.1g Carbs: 21.1g Protein: 3.2g Fiber: 2.9g

Noodle and Rice Pilaf

Preparation Time: 5 minutes

Cooking Time: 33 to 44 minutes

Servings: 6 to 8

Ingredients:

- 1 cup whole-wheat noodles, broken into 1/8 inch pieces
- 2 cups long-grain brown rice
- 6½ cups low-sodium vegetable broth
- 1 teaspoon ground cumin
- ½ teaspoon dried oregano

Directions:

1. Combine the noodles and rice in a saucepan over medium heat and cook for 3 to 4 minutes, or until they begin to smell toasted.

2. Stir in the vegetable broth, cumin and oregano. Bring to a boil. Reduce the heat to medium-low. Cover and cook for 30 to 40 minutes, or until all water is absorbed.

Nutrition: Calories: 287 Fat: 2.5g Carbs: 58.1g
Protein: 7.9g Fiber: 5.0g

Easy Millet Loaf

Preparation Time: 5 minutes

Cooking Time: 1 hour 15 minutes

Servings: 4

Ingredients:

- 1¼ cups millet
- 4 cups unsweetened tomato juice
- 1 medium onion, chopped
- 1 to 2 cloves garlic
- ½ teaspoon dried sage
- ½ teaspoon dried basil
- ½ teaspoon poultry seasoning

Directions:

1. Preheat the oven to 350ºF (180ºC).

2. Place the millet in a large bowl.

3. Place the remaining ingredients in a blender and pulse until smooth. Add to the bowl with the millet and mix well.

4. Pour the mixture into a shallow casserole dish. Cover and bake in the oven for 1¼ hours, or until set.

5. Serve warm.

Nutrition: Calories: 315 Fat: 3.4g Carbs: 61.6g Protein: 10.2g Fiber: 9.6g

Walnut-Oat Burgers

Preparation Time: 5 minutes

Cooking Time: 20 to 30 minutes

Servings: 6 to 8

Ingredients:

- 1 medium onion, finely chopped
- 2 cups rolled oats
- 2 cups unsweetened low-fat soy milk
- 1 cup finely chopped walnuts
- 1 tablespoon soy sauce
- ½ teaspoon dried sage
- ½ teaspoon garlic powder
- ½ teaspoon onion powder
- ½ teaspoon dried thyme
- ¼ teaspoon dried marjoram

Directions:

1. Stir together all the ingredients in a large bowl. Let rest for 20 minutes.
2. Form the mixture into six or eight patties. Cook the patties on a nonstick griddle over

medium heat for 20 to 30 minutes, or until browned on each side.

3. Serve warm.

Nutrition: Calories: 341 Fat: 13.9g Carbs: 42.4g Protein: 13.9g Fiber: 6.8g

Spicy Beans and Rice

Preparation Time: 5 minutes

Cooking Time: 45 minutes

Servings: 4 to 6

Ingredients:

- 1½ cups long-grain brown rice
- 1 (19-ounce / 539-g) can kidney beans, rinsed and drained
- 2 cups chopped onion
- 1 cup mild salsa
- 1 teaspoon ground cumin
- 16 ounces (454 g) tomatoes, chopped
- 3 cups water

Directions:

1. In a pot, bring the water to a boil. Stir in the rice. Bring to a boil again and stir in the remaining ingredients, except for the tomatoes. Return to a boil. Reduce the heat to low. Cover and simmer for 45 minutes.

2. Remove from the heat and stir in the tomatoes. Let sit for 5 minutes, covered.

Nutrition: Calories: 386 Fat: 7.1g Carbs: 71.1g Protein: 11.1g Fiber: 5.8g

Black-Eyed Peas and Corn Salad

Preparation Time: 30 minutes

Cooking Time: 50 minutes

Servings: 4

Ingredients:

- 2½ cups cooked black-eyed peas
- 3 ears corn, kernels removed
- 1 medium ripe tomato, diced
- ½ medium red onion, peeled and diced small
- ½ red bell pepper, deseeded and diced small
- 1 jalapeño pepper, deseeded and minced
- ½ cup finely chopped cilantro
- ¼ cup plus 2 tablespoons balsamic vinegar
- 3 cloves garlic, peeled and minced
- 1 teaspoon toasted and ground cumin seeds

Directions:

1. Stir together all the ingredients in a large bowl and refrigerate for about 1 hour, or until well chilled.
2. Serve chilled.

Nutrition: Calories: 247 Fat: 1.8g Carbs: 47.6g

Protein: 12.9g Fiber: 11.7g

Indian Tomato and Garbanzo Stew

Preparation Time: 15 minutes

Cooking Time: 50 minutes

Servings: 4 to 6

Ingredients:

- 1 large onion, quartered and thinly sliced
- 1 inch fresh ginger, peeled and minced
- 2 cloves garlic, peeled and minced
- 1 teaspoon curry powder
- 1 teaspoon cumin seeds
- 1 teaspoon black mustard seeds
- 1 teaspoon coriander seeds,
- 1½ pounds (680 g) tomatoes, deseeded and puréed
- 1 red bell pepper, cut into ½-inch dice
- 1 green bell pepper, cut into ½-inch dice
- 3 cups cooked garbanzo beans
- 1 tablespoon garam masala
- 1/3 cup water

Directions:

1. Heat the water in a medium saucepan over medium-low heat. Add the onion, ginger, garlic, curry powder, and seeds to the pan. Sauté for about 10 minutes, or until the onion is tender, stirring frequently.

2. Add the tomatoes and simmer, uncovered, for 10 minutes. Add the peppers and garbanzo beans. Reduce the heat. Cover and simmer for 30 minutes, stirring occasionally. Stir in the garam masala and serve.

Nutrition: Calories: 100 Fat: 1.2g Carbs: 20.9g Protein: 5.1g Fiber: 7.0g

Simple Baked Navy Beans

Preparation Time: 10 minutes

Cooking Time: 2½ to 3 hours

Servings: 8

Ingredients:

- 1½ cups navy beans
- 8 cups water
- 1 bay leaf
- ½ cup finely chopped green bell pepper
- ½ cup finely chopped onion
- 1 teaspoon minced garlic
- ½ cup unsweetened tomato purée
- 3 tablespoons molasses
- 1 tablespoon fresh lemon juice

Directions:

1. Preheat the oven to 300ºF (150ºC).

2. Place the beans and water in a large pot, along with the bay leaf, green pepper, onion and garlic. Cover and cook for 1½ to 2 hours, or until the beans are softened. Remove from the heat

and drain, reserving the cooking liquid. Discard the bay leaf.

3. Transfer the mixture to a casserole dish with a cover. Stir in the remaining ingredients and 1 cup of the reserved cooking liquid. Bake in the oven for 1 hour, covered. Stir occasionally during baking and add a little more cooking liquid if needed to keep the beans moist.

4. Serve warm.

Nutrition: Calories: 162 Fat: 0.6g Carbs: 31.3g Protein: 9.1g Fiber: 6.4g

Vinegary Black Beans

Preparation Time: 10 minutes

Cooking Time: 2 hours

Servings: 8

Ingredients:

- 1 pound (454 g) black beans, soaked overnight and drained
- 10½ cups water, divided
- 1 green bell pepper, cut in half
- 1 onion, finely chopped
- 1 green bell pepper, finely chopped
- 4 cloves garlic, pressed
- 1 tablespoon maple syrup (optional)
- 1 tablespoon Mrs. Dash seasoning
- 1 bay leaf
- ¼ teaspoon dried oregano
- 2 tablespoons cider vinegar

Directions:

1. Place the beans, 10 cups of the water, and green bell pepper in a large pot. Cook over medium heat for about 45 minutes, or until the green

pepper is tendered. Remove the green pepper and discard.

2. Meanwhile, in a different pot, combine the onion, chopped green pepper, garlic and the remaining ½ cup of the water. Sauté for 15 to 20 minutes, or until soft.

3. Add 1 cup of the cooked beans to the pot with vegetables. Mash the beans and vegetables with a potato masher. Add to the pot with the beans, along with the maple syrup (if desired), Mrs. Dash, bay leaf and oregano. Cover and cook over low heat for 1 hour.

4. Drizzle in the vinegar and continue to cook for another hour.

5. Serve warm.

Nutrition: Calories: 226 Fat: 0.9g Carbs: 42.7g Protein: 12.9g Fiber: 9.9g

Spiced Lentil Burgers

Preparation Time: 10 minutes

Cooking Time: 43 minutes

Servings: 4

Ingredients:

- ¼ cup minced onion
- 1 clove garlic, minced
- 2 tablespoons water
- 1 cup chopped boiled potatoes
- 1 cup cooked lentils
- 2 tablespoons minced fresh parsley
- 1 teaspoon onion powder
- 1 teaspoon minced fresh basil
- 1 teaspoon dried dill
- 1 teaspoon paprika

Directions:

1. Preheat the oven to 350ºF (180ºC).

2. In a pot, sauté the onion and garlic in the water for about 3 minutes, or until soft.

3. Combine the lentils and potatoes in a large bowl and mash together well. Add the cooked onion

and garlic along with the remaining ingredients to the lentil-potato mixture and stir until well combined.

4. Form the mixture into four patties and place on a nonstick baking sheet. Bake in the oven for 20 minutes. Turnover and bake for an additional 20 minutes.

5. Serve hot.

Nutrition: Calories: 101 Fat: 0.4g Carbs: 19.9g Protein: 5.5g Fiber: 5.3g

Pecan-Maple Granola

Preparation Time: 5 minutes

Cooking Time: 50 minutes

Servings: 4

Ingredients:

- 1½ cups rolled oats
- ¼ cup maple syrup (optional)
- ¼ cup pecan pieces
- 1 teaspoon vanilla extract
- ½ teaspoon ground cinnamon

Directions:

1. Preheat the oven to 300ºF (150ºC). Line a baking sheet with parchment paper.
2. In a large bowl, stir together all the ingredients until the oats and pecan pieces are completely coated.
3. Spread the mixture on the baking sheet in an even layer. Bake in the oven for 20 minutes, stirring once halfway through cooking.
4. Remove from the oven and allow to cool on the countertop for 30 minutes before serving.

Nutrition: Calories: 221 Fat: 17.2g Carbs: 5.1g

Protein: 4.9g Fiber: 3.8g

Bean and Summer Squash Sauté

Preparation Time: 10 minutes

Cooking Time: 15 to 16 minutes

Servings: 4

Ingredients:

- 1 medium red onion, peeled and thinly sliced
- 4 yellow squash, cut into ½-inch rounds
- 4 medium zucchinis, cut into ½-inch rounds
- 1 (15-ounce / 425-g) can navy beans, drained and rinsed
- 2 cups corn kernels
- Zest of 2 lemons
- 1 cup finely chopped basil
- Salt, to taste (optional)
- Freshly ground black pepper, to taste

Directions:

1. Place the onion in a large saucepan and sauté over medium heat for 7 to 8 minutes. Add water 1 to 2 tablespoons at a time to keep the onion from sticking to the pan.

---

2. Add the squash, zucchini, beans, and corn and cook for about 8 minutes, or until the squash is softened.
3. Remove from the heat. Stir in the lemon zest and basil. Season with salt (if desired) and pepper.
4. Serve hot.

Nutrition: Calories: 298 Fat: 2.2g Carbs: 60.4g Protein: 17.2g Fiber: 13.6g

Peppery Black Beans

Preparation Time: 10 minutes

Cooking Time: 33 to 34 minutes

Servings: 4

Ingredients:

- 1 red bell pepper, deseeded and chopped
- 1 medium yellow onion, peeled and chopped
- 2 jalapeño peppers, deseeded and minced
- 4 cloves garlic, peeled and minced
- 1 tablespoon thyme
- 1 tablespoon curry powder
- 1½ teaspoons ground allspice
- 1 teaspoon freshly ground black pepper
- 1 (15-ounce / 425-g)can diced tomatoes
- 4 cups cooked black beans

Directions:

1. Add the red bell pepper and onion to a saucepan and sauté over medium heat for 10 minutes, or until the onion is softened. Add water 1 to 2 tablespoons at a time to keep the vegetables from sticking to the pan.

2. Stir in the jalapeño peppers, garlic, thyme, curry powder, allspice and black pepper. Cook for 3 to 4 minutes, then add the tomatoes and black beans. Cook over medium heat for 20 minutes, covered.
3. Serve immediately.

Nutrition: Calories: 283 Fat: 1.7g Carbs: 52.8g Protein: 17.4g Fiber: 19.8g

Walnut, Coconut, and Oat Granola

Preparation Time: 15 minutes

Cooking Time: 1 hour 40 minutes

Servings: 4

Ingredients:

- 1 cup chopped walnuts
- 1 cup unsweetened, shredded coconut
- 2 cups rolled oats
- 1 teaspoon ground cinnamon
- 2 tablespoons hemp seeds
- 2 tablespoons ground flaxseeds
- 2 tablespoons chia seeds
- ¾ teaspoon salt (optional)
- ¼ cup maple syrup
- ¼ cup water
- 1 teaspoon vanilla extract
- ½ cup dried cranberries

Directions:

1. Preheat the oven to 250ºF (120ºC). Line a baking sheet with parchment paper.

2. Mix the walnuts, coconut, rolled oats, cinnamon, hemp seeds, flaxseeds, chia seeds, and salt (if desired) in a bowl.

3. Combine the maple syrup and water in a saucepan. Bring to a boil over medium heat, then pour in the bowl of walnut mixture.

4. Add the vanilla extract to the bowl of mixture. Stir to mix well. Pour the mixture in the baking sheet, then level with a spatula so the mixture coat the bottom evenly.

5. Place the baking sheet in the preheated oven and bake for 90 minutes or until browned and crispy. Stir the mixture every 15 minutes.

6. Remove the baking sheet from the oven. Allow to cool for 10 minutes, then serve with dried cranberries on top.

Nutrition: Calories: 1870 Fat: 115.8g Carbs: 238.0g Protein: 59.8g Fiber: 68.9g

Ritzy Fava Bean Ratatouille

Preparation Time: 15 minutes

Cooking Time: 40 minutes

Servings: 4

Ingredients:

- 1 medium red onion, peeled and thinly sliced
- 2 tablespoons low-sodium vegetable broth
- 1 large eggplant, stemmed and cut into ½-inch dice
- 1 red bell pepper, seeded and diced
- 2 cups cooked fava beans
- 2 Roma tomatoes, chopped
- 1 medium zucchini, diced
- 2 cloves garlic, peeled and finely chopped
- ¼ cup finely chopped basil
- Salt, to taste (optional)
- Ground black pepper, to taste

Directions:

1. Add the onion to a saucepan and sauté for 7 minutes or until caramelized.

2. Add the vegetable broth, eggplant and red bell pepper to the pan and sauté for 10 more minutes.

3. Add the fava beans, tomatoes, zucchini, and garlic to the pan and sauté for an additional 5 minutes.

4. Reduce the heat to medium-low. Put the pan lid on and cook for 15 minutes or until the vegetables are soft. Stir the vegetables halfway through.

5. Transfer them onto a large serving plate. Sprinkle with basil, salt (if desired), and black pepper before serving.

Nutrition: Calories: 114 Fat: 1.0g Carbs: 24.2g Protein: 7.4g Fiber: 10.3g

Peppers and Black Beans with Brown Rice

Preparation Time: 15 minutes

Cooking Time: 20 minutes

Servings: 4

Ingredients:

- 2 jalapeño peppers, diced
- 1 red bell pepper, seeded and diced
- 1 medium yellow onion, peeled and diced
- 2 tablespoons low-sodium vegetable broth
- 1 teaspoon toasted and ground cumin seeds
- 1½ teaspoons toasted oregano
- 5 cloves garlic, peeled and minced
- 4 cups cooked black beans
- Salt, to taste (optional)
- Ground black pepper, to taste
- 3 cups cooked brown rice
- 1 lime, quartered
- 1 cup chopped cilantro

Directions:

1. Add the jalapeño peppers, bell pepper, and onion to a saucepan and sauté for 7 minutes or until the onion is well browned and caramelized.

2. Add vegetable broth, cumin, oregano, and garlic to the pan and sauté for 3 minutes or until fragrant.

3. Add the black beans and sauté for 10 minutes or until the vegetables are tender. Sprinkle with salt (if desired) and black pepper halfway through.

4. Arrange the brown rice on a platter, then top with the cooked vegetables. Garnish with lime wedges and cilantro before serving.

Nutrition: Calories: 426 Fat: 2.6g Carbs: 82.4g Protein: 20.2g Fiber: 19.5g

Black-Eyed Pea, Beet, and Carrot Stew

Preparation Time: 15 minutes

Cooking Time: 40 minutes

Servings: 2

Ingredients:

- ½ cup black-eyed peas, soaked in water overnight
- 3 cups water
- 1 large beet, peeled and cut into ½-inch pieces (about ¾ cup)
- 1 large carrot, peeled and cut into ½-inch pieces (about ¾ cup)
- ¼ teaspoon turmeric
- ¼ teaspoon toasted and ground cumin seeds
- 1/8 teaspoon asafetida
- ¼ cup finely chopped parsley
- ¼ teaspoon cayenne pepper
- ¼ teaspoon salt (optional)
- ½ teaspoon fresh lime juice

Directions:

1. Pour the black-eyed peas and water in a pot, then cook over medium heat for 25 minutes.
2. Add the beet and carrot to the pot and cook for 10 more minutes. Add more water if necessary.
3. Add the turmeric, cumin, asafetida, parsley, and cayenne pepper to the pot and cook for an additional 6 minutes or until the vegetables are soft. Stir the mixture periodically. Sprinkle with salt, if desired.
4. Drizzle the lime juice on top before serving in a large bowl.

Nutrition: Calories: 84 | fat: 0.7g | carbs: 16.6g | protein: 4.1g | fiber: 4.5g

Koshari

Preparation Time: 15 minutes

Cooking Time: 2 hours 10 minutes

Servings: 6

Ingredients:

- 1 cup green lentils, rinsed
- 3 cups water
- Salt, to taste (optional)
- 1 large onion, peeled and minced
- 2 tablespoons low-sodium vegetable broth
- 4 cloves garlic, peeled and minced
- ½ teaspoon ground allspice
- 1 teaspoon ground coriander
- 1 teaspoon ground cumin
- 2 tablespoons tomato paste
- ½ teaspoon crushed red pepper flakes
- 3 large tomatoes, diced
- 1 cup cooked medium-grain brown rice
- 1 cup whole-grain elbow macaroni, cooked, drained, and kept warm
- 1 tablespoon brown rice vinegar

Directions:

1. Put the lentils and water in a saucepan, and sprinkle with salt, if desired. Bring to a boil over high heat. Reduce the heat to medium, then put the pan lid on and cook for 45 minutes or until the water is mostly absorbed. Pour the cooked lentils in the bowl and set aside.
2. Add the onion to a nonstick skillet, then sauté over medium heat for 15 minutes or until caramelized.
3. Add vegetable broth and garlic to the skillet and sauté for 3 minutes or until fragrant.
4. Add the allspice, coriander, cumin, tomato paste, and red pepper flakes to the skillet and sauté for an additional 3 minutes until aromatic.
5. Add the tomatoes to the skillet and sauté for 15 minutes or until the tomatoes are wilted. Sprinkle with salt, if desired.
6. Arrange the cooked brown rice on the bottom of a large platter, then top the rice with macaroni, and then spread the lentils over. Pour the tomato mixture and brown rice vinegar over before serving.

Nutrition: Calories: 201 Fat: 1.6g Carbs: 41.8g

Protein: 6.5g Fiber: 3.6g

DRINKS

Chocolatey Banana Shake

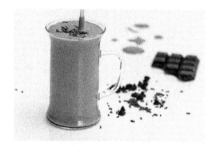

Preparation Time: 10 minutes

Cooking Time: 10 minutes

Servings: 2

Ingredients:

- 2 medium frozen bananas, peeled
- 4 dates, pitted
- 4 tablespoons peanut butter
- 4 tablespoons rolled oats
- 2 tablespoons cacao powder
- 2 tablespoons chia seeds
- 2 cups unsweetened soymilk

Directions:

1. Place all the ingredients in a high-speed blender and pulse until creamy.
2. Pour into two glasses and serve immediately.

Nutrition: Calories: 502 Fat: 4g Protein: 11g

Sugar: 9g

Fruity Tofu Smoothie

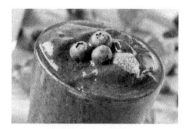

Preparation Time: 10 minutes

Cooking Time: 10 minutes

Servings: 2

Ingredients:

- 12 ounces silken tofu, pressed and drained
- 2 medium bananas, peeled
- 1½ cups fresh blueberries
- 1 tablespoon maple syrup
- 1½ cups unsweetened soymilk
- ¼ cup ice cubes

Directions:

1. Place all the ingredients in a high-speed blender and pulse until creamy.
2. Pour into two glasses and serve immediately.

Nutrition: Calories 235 Carbohydrates: 1.9g
Protein: 14.3g Fat: 18.9g

Green Fruity Smoothie

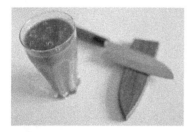

Preparation Time: 10 minutes

Cooking Time: 10 minutes

Servings: 2

Ingredients:

- 1 cup frozen mango, peeled, pitted, and chopped
- 1 large frozen banana, peeled
- 2 cups fresh baby spinach
- 1 scoop unsweetened vegan vanilla protein powder
- ¼ cup pumpkin seeds
- 2 tablespoons hemp hearts
- 1½ cups unsweetened almond milk

Directions:

1. In a high-speed blender, place all the ingredients and pulse until creamy.
2. Pour into two glasses and serve immediately.

Nutrition: Calories 206 Carbohydrates: 1.3g

Protein: 23.5g Fat: 11.9g

Protein Latte

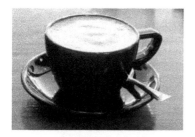

Preparation Time: 10 minutes

Cooking Time: 10 minutes

Servings: 2

Ingredients:

- 2 cups hot brewed coffee
- 1¼ cups coconut milk
- 2 teaspoons coconut oil
- 2 scoops unsweetened vegan vanilla protein powder

Directions:

1. Place all the ingredients in a high-speed blender and pulse until creamy.
2. Pour into two serving mugs and serve immediately.

Nutrition: Calories 483 Carbs: 5.2g Protein: 45.2g Fat: 31.2g

Health Boosting Juices

Preparation Time: 10 minutes

Cooking Time: 15 minutes

Servings: 2

Ingredients for a red juice:

- 4 beetroots, quartered
- 2 cups of strawberries
- 2 cups of blueberries
- Ingredients for an orange juice:
- 4 green or red apples, halved
- 10 carrots
- ½ lemon, peeled
- 1" of ginger
- Ingredients for a yellow juice:
- 2 green or red apples, quartered
- 4 oranges, peeled and halved
- ½ lemon, peeled
- 1" of ginger
- Ingredients for a lime juice:
- 6 stalks of celery
- 1 cucumber
- 2 green apples, quartered

- 2 pears, quartered

- Ingredients for a green juice:

- ½ a pineapple, peeled and sliced

- 8 leaves of kale

- 2 fresh bananas, peeled

Directions:

1. Juice all ingredients in a juicer, chill and serve.

Nutrition: Calories 316 Carbs: 13.5g Protein: 37.8g Fat: 12.2g

Thai Iced Tea

Preparation Time: 5 minutes

Cooking Time: 10 minutes

Servings: 4

Ingredients:

- 4 cups of water
- 1 can of light coconut milk (14 oz.)
- ¼ cup of maple syrup
- ¼ cup of muscovado sugar
- 1 teaspoon of vanilla extract
- 2 tablespoons of loose-leaf black tea

Directions:

1. In a large saucepan, over medium heat bring the water to a boil.
2. Turn off the heat and add in the tea, cover and let steep for five minutes.
3. Strain the tea into a bowl or jug. Add the maple syrup, muscovado sugar, and vanilla extract. Give it a good whisk to blend all the ingredients together.

4. Set in the refrigerator to chill. Upon serving, pour ¾ of the tea into each glass, top with coconut milk and stir.

Tips:

Add a shot of dark rum to turn this iced tea into a cocktail.

You could substitute the coconut milk for almond or rice milk too.

Nutrition: Calories 844 Carbohydrates: 2.3g Protein: 21.6g Fat: 83.1g

Hot Chocolate

Preparation Time: 5 minutes

Cooking Time: 15 minutes

Servings: 2

Ingredients:

- Pinch of brown sugar
- 2 cups of milk, soy or almond, unsweetened
- 2 tablespoons of cocoa powder
- ½ cup of vegan chocolate

Directions:

1. In a medium saucepan, over medium heat gently bring the milk to a boil. Whisk in the cocoa powder.
2. Remove from the heat, add a pinch of sugar and chocolate. Give it a good stir until smooth, serve and enjoy.

Tips:

You may substitute the almond or soy milk for coconut milk too.

Nutrition: Calories 452 Carbs: 29.8g Protein: 15.2g Fat: 30.2g

Chai and Chocolate Milkshake

Preparation Time: 5 minutes

Cooking Time: 15 minutes

Servings: 2 servings

Ingredients:

- 1 and ½ cups of almond milk, sweetened or unsweetened
- 3 bananas, peeled and frozen 12 hours before use
- 4 dates, pitted
- 1 and ½ teaspoons of chocolate powder, sweetened or unsweetened
- ½ teaspoon of vanilla extract
- ½ teaspoon of cinnamon
- ¼ teaspoon of ground ginger
- Pinch of ground cardamom
- Pinch of ground cloves
- Pinch of ground nutmeg
- ½ cup of ice cubes

Directions:

1. Add all the ingredients to a blender except for the ice-cubes. Pulse until smooth and creamy, add the ice-cubes, pulse a few more times and serve.

Tips:

The dates provide enough sweetness to the recipe, however, you are welcome to add maple syrup or honey for a sweeter drink.

Nutrition: Calories 452 Carbs: 29.8g Protein: 15.2g Fat: 30.2g

Colorful Infused Water

Preparation Time: 5 minutes

Cooking Time: 1 hour

Servings: 8 servings

Ingredients:

- 1 cup of strawberries, fresh or frozen
- 1 cup of blueberries, fresh or frozen
- 1 tablespoon of baobab powder
- 1 cup of ice cubes
- 4 cups of sparkling water

Directions:

2. In a large water jug, add in the sparkling water, ice cubes, and baobab powder. Give it a good stir.

3. Add in the strawberries and blueberries and cover the infused water, store in the refrigerator for one hour before serving.

Tips:

Store for 12 hours for optimum taste and nutritional benefits.

Instead of using strawberries and blueberries, add slices of lemon and six mint leaves, one cup of mangoes or cherries, or half a cup of leafy greens such as kale and/or spinach.

Nutrition: Calories 163 Carbs: 4.1g Protein: 1.7g Fat: 15.5g

Hibiscus Tea

Preparation Time: 1 Minute

Cooking Time: 5 minutes

Servings: 2 servings

Ingredients:

- 1 tablespoon of raisins, diced
- 6 Almonds, raw and unsalted
- ½ teaspoon of hibiscus powder
- 2 cups of water

Directions:

1. Bring the water to a boil in a small saucepan, add in the hibiscus powder and raisins. Give it a good stir, cover and let simmer for a further two minutes.

2. Strain into a teapot and serve with a side helping of almonds.

Tips:

As an alternative to this tea, do not strain it and serve with the raisin pieces still swirling around in the teacup.

You could also serve this tea chilled for those hotter days.

Double or triple the recipe to provide you with iced-tea to enjoy during the week without having to make a fresh pot each time.

Nutrition: Calories 139 Carbohydrates: 2.7g Protein: 8.7g Fat: 10.3

Lemon and Rosemary Iced Tea

Preparation Time: 5 minutes

Cooking Time: 10 minutes

Servings: 4 servings

Ingredients:

- 4 cups of water
- 4 earl grey tea bags
- ¼ cup of sugar
- 2 lemons
- 1 sprig of rosemary

Directions:

1. Peel the two lemons and set the fruit aside.
2. In a medium saucepan, over medium heat combine the water, sugar, and lemon peels. Bring this to a boil.
3. Remove from the heat and place the rosemary and tea into the mixture. Cover the saucepan and steep for five minutes.
4. Add the juice of the two peeled lemons to the mixture, strain, chill, and serve.

Tips: Skip the sugar and use honey to taste.

Do not squeeze the tea bags as they can cause the tea to become bitter.

Nutrition: Calories 229 Carbs: 33.2g Protein: 31.1g Fat: 10.2g

Lavender and Mint Iced Tea

Preparation Time: 5 minutes

Cooking Time: 10 minutes

Servings: 8 servings

Ingredients:

- 8 cups of water
- 1/3 cup of dried lavender buds
- ¼ cup of mint

Directions:

1. Add the mint and lavender to a pot and set this aside.
2. Add in eight cups of boiling water to the pot. Sweeten to taste, cover and let steep for ten minutes. Strain, chill, and serve.

Tips:

Use a sweetener of your choice when making this iced tea.

Add spirits to turn this iced tea into a summer cocktail.

Nutrition: Calories 266 Carbs: 9.3g Protein: 20.9g Fat: 16.1g

Conclusion

Vegan recipes do not need to be boring. There are so many different combinations of veggies, fruits, whole grains, beans, seeds, and nuts that you will be able to make unique meal plans for many months. These recipes contain the instructions along with the necessary ingredients and nutritional information.

If you ever come across someone complaining that they can't follow the plant-based diet because it's expensive, hard to cater for, lacking in variety, or tasteless, feel free to have them take a look at this book. In no time, you'll have another companion walking beside you on this road to healthier eating and better living.

Although healthy, many people are still hesitant to give vegan food a try. They mistakenly believe that these would be boring, tasteless, and complicated to make. This is the farthest thing from the truth.

Fruits and vegetables are organically delicious, fragrant, and vibrantly colored. If you add herbs, mushrooms, and nuts to the mix, dishes will always come out packed full of flavor it only takes a bit of effort and time to prepare great-tasting vegan meals for your family.

How easy was that? Don't we all want a seamless and easy way to cook like this?

I believe cooking is taking a better turn and the days, when we needed so many ingredients to provide a decent meal, were gone. Now, with easy tweaks, we can make delicious, quick, and easy meals. Most importantly, we get to save a bunch of cash on groceries.

I am grateful for downloading this book and taking the time to read it. I know that you have learned a lot and you had a great time reading it. Writing books is the best way to share the skills I have with your and the best tips too.

I know that there are many books and choosing my book is amazing. I am thankful that you stopped and took time to decide. You made a great decision and I am sure that you enjoyed it.

I will be even happier if you will add some comments. Feedbacks helped by growing and they still do. They help me to choose better content and new ideas. So, maybe your feedback can trigger an idea for my next book.

Hopefully, this book has helped you understand that vegetarian recipes and diet can improve your life, not only by improving your health and helping you lose weight, but also by saving you money and time. I sincerely hope that the recipes provided in this book have proven to be quick, easy, and delicious, and have provided you with enough variety to keep your taste buds interested and curious.

I hope you enjoyed reading about my book!

CPSIA information can be obtained
at www.ICGtesting.com
Printed in the USA
LVHW051627010621
689061LV00002B/513